20 Awesome Raw Desserts You Can't Live Without

Recipes 4 Raw Food

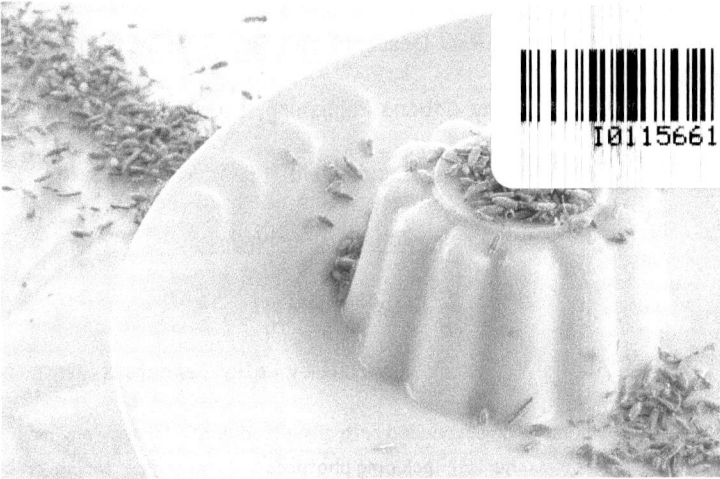

A collection of 20 raw desserts that are fun, easy, and nutritious!

Raw Food Recipes for a Healthy Lifestyle

By Kathy Tennefoss

Member of the Raw Foods Association

RECIPES 4
RAW FOOD

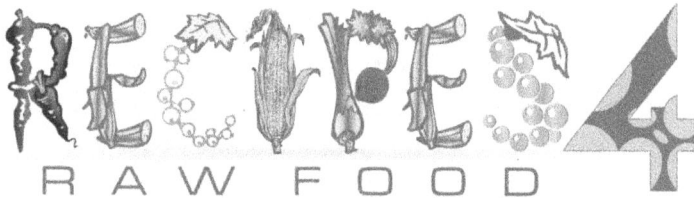

820 Awesome Raw Desserts You Can't Live Without

Sunny Cabana Publishing, L.L.C.

Fort Lauderdale, FL

www.sunnycabanapublishing.com

By Kathy Tennefoss

Published by Kathleen Tennefoss
Printed in the United States of America
Author: Kathy Tennefoss
Editor: Shawn M Tennefoss
13-digit ISBN: 9781936874088
10-digit ISBN: 1936874083
SECOND EDITION
Library of Congress Cataloging-in-Publication Data has been applied for

This book is dedicated to My dad James Kelley for pushing me in the right direction regarding healthy eating, living a healthy active life, and to my loving husband Shawn Tennefoss for suffering through my computer difficulties and taking the time to show me how to orchestrate this book along with sharing his life and journey with me.

Cover Design: Kathy & Shawn Tennefoss

Second Edition, 2011

Acknowledgements:

Thanks to everyone who encouraged and inspired me and gave me excellent input and feedback in the raw food industry, including my sister Heather McNerney, my husband Shawn M Tennefoss, my father James Kelley, and Melissa Hernandez and her wonderful family! Without everyone's input I would not have finished this book or started other raw food recipe books. I am extremely grateful to everyone.

Please feel free to email suggestions, comments, or corrections to recipes4rawfood@yahoo.com.

Disclaimer:
The responsibility for any adverse detoxification effects resulting from using these recipes described lies not with the author or distributors of this book. This book is not intended for medical advice just as suggestion.
Please enjoy these recipes with your friends and family.

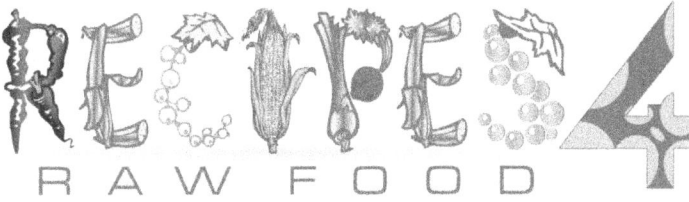

RECIPES 4
RAW FOOD

Table of Contents

Intro

Today you hear "I'm too busy and I don't have time to eat healthy or it costs too much". Well I'm here to say that it only takes a few minutes to have a healthy meal. For the time it takes to go to the drive through and wait in line to have some high fat low nutrition meal you can make a quick raw meal. If cost is your concern buy your organic produce in bulk or choose an organic buying club that delivers produce weekly to your home. You don't have to eat this way everyday but you will feel a huge difference in your body just after a few days of eating this way. Your skin will start to feel better, your clothes will be fitting loser, and you might even have more energy! Isn't that worth it!

Don't let the title of this book scare you. You can have your dessert and eat it too without gaining weight or having high cholesterol. I want to show you how easy and fun it is to have healthy desserts. Desserts always get a bad name but not anymore! You can create great healthy desserts for you and your whole family with these easy to follow recipes!

Please try to use as much organic produce as possible when making your desserts or any other meal you plan to prepare. Starting with the freshest ingredients is always the best option plus they taste better and you're helping the environment by purchasing local organic ingredients.

APPLE TARTLETS with CACAO BANANA SAUCE

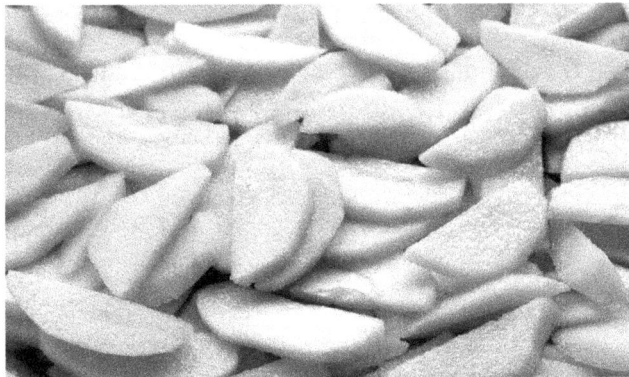

Serves 4

Crust:

3 cups young coconut, shredded & dehydrated
3 medjool dates (pitted)

Blend coconut in blender or food processor until fine and then add the dates and blend. Press into 4, 3 inch tartlet pans, lined with parchment paper. Freeze for 2 hours. Take out, discard liner, and let stand for 15 minutes before adding filling.

Filling:

4 cups apples, cored & peeled
$\frac{1}{2}$ Cup of Chopped Raw Almonds
1 tsp cinnamon

1/8 tsp nutmeg
1/4 tsp fresh ginger
2 tbsp lemon juice

Put apples in a food processor until chunky. Stir in lemon juice and spices. Pour into crust and top with chopped almond sauce.

Cacao Banana Sauce:

1 Half of Banana
2 tsp of raw Cacao powder
1 Young coconut
2 fresh medjool date

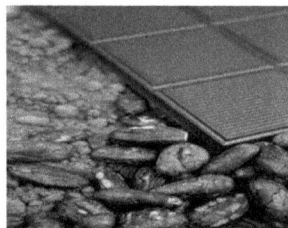

Carefully open up young coconuts and empty liquid into a Vita mixer blender. Scoop out white "meat" out of the coconut and put into blender as well. Add half of the banana, pitted dates, and cocoa powder into blender, blend until smooth.

Place tartlet on plate, spoon sauce on tartlet, and sprinkle chopped almonds on top.

Lemon Cookies

2 cups raw cashews (not soaked)
2 cups shredded coconut
½ cup lemon juice
¼ Cup of almond milk
1/4 cup lemon zest
1/4 cup maple syrup

Blend all ingredients in a food processor until smooth and then form into cookie shapes and dehydrate for 12hours at 90 degrees.

Coconut Haystacks

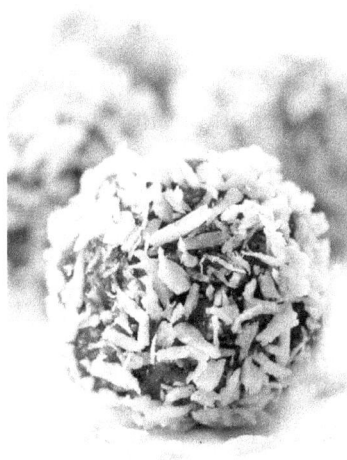

1 Cup coconut oil
½ Cup raw honey
¼ Cup maple syrup
½ Cup cocoa powder
1 teaspoon vanilla extract
4 Cups shredded coconut

Blend all ingredients except the shredded coconut in a food processor until smooth. Next add the coconut to the mixture and form into round balls and place on parchment paper and freeze. They will become soft if left out of the freezer for very long so bring them out around 15 minutes before serving.

Cherry Crisp

Yield: 1 (8-inch) crisp

Crumble Topping:
2 cups raw walnuts or pecans chopped
$\frac{1}{2}$ cup raw oats
1/2 cup unsweetened shredded dried coconut
1/4 teaspoon ground cinnamon
1/4teaspoon ground nutmeg
1/4 teaspoon salt
1/2 cup dried cherries chopped
8 pitted medjool dates ground up small
1/4 cup maple syrup

Filling:
30 oz of frozen cherries frozen thawed and drained
3/4cup pitted medjool dates, soaked
1 tablespoon fresh lemon juice

Blend all of the filling and put into a glass baking container. Then take the crumble topping and mix by hand until smooth and then put the crumble on top of the cherries.

Raw Key Lime Pudding

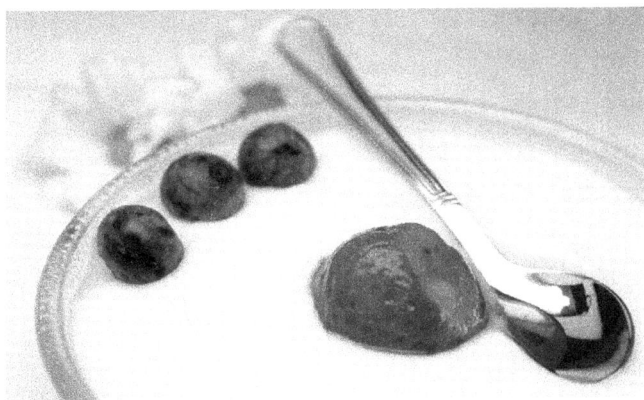

1 cup young coconut meat
2 tablespoons coconut butter
$\frac{1}{2}$ cup macadamia nuts
$\frac{1}{4}$ cup coconut water
4 tablespoons key lime juice
1 key lime for zesting
$\frac{1}{4}$ teaspoon Celtic sea salt
1 Tablespoon of maple syrup

Mix the macadamia nuts, water, coconut water and lime juice in a high-powered blender, vita mixer, or food processor and blend until smooth. Then add all other ingredients and blend until smooth. Refrigerate for at least 1 hour before serving so that pudding may thicken. Then top with key lime zest.

Almond Butter Bars

3/4 cup raw almond butter
1/4 cup Macadamia nut butter
1/2 cup raw honey
1 cup raw sesame seeds
1/4 cup of raw cacao powder
1/2 cup of shredded coconut

Mix all ingredients in a food processor on slow and then remove and put into a glass pan and then top with chopped raw almonds!

Apricot Cookies

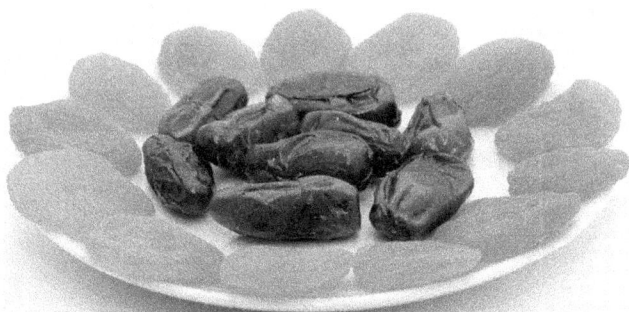

2 Cups oats soaked
2 Cups dried apricots
1 Cup of dates pitted
½ Cup dried figs soaked
1 Cup finely ground flaxseeds
1 Cup pecans chopped
½ Cup maple syrup
(Save the water from soaking the figs)

In a vita mixer add the oats, dates, dried figs; soak water, finely ground flaxseeds, and maple syrup. Take the mixture and add the chopped apricots and chopped pecans and form into cookies and dehydrate for 100 degrees for 4 hours on each side.

Raw Pumpkin Pie

Crust:
1 Cup raw pecans ground up fine
1 Tbsp. lemon zest
6 dates pitted
Mix all ingredients in a food processor until smooth and then spread out evenly in dish.

Filling

2 Cups Raw Pumpkin cut up
1 Avocado pitted

1 Tbsp Lemon Juice
2 Teaspoons of pumpkin spices
2 Tablespoons of maple syrup
2 Tablespoon of finely ground flaxseeds
1/2 Teaspoon Fresh Ginger

Put all ingredients in food processor and process until smooth. Put into dish onto crust and spread evenly. Set in Fridge to allow to set some more. Serve with following whip.

Whip:

1 Cup of Macadamia Nuts
7 Pitted Dates
1 Tbsp. Lemon Juice
2-3 Tablespoons of orange juice

Put all ingredients in Blender and let process until smooth. Keep adding the orange juice to keep the mixture thin enough to whip in the blender.

You want the whip to be smooth and thick but loose enough to just about pour.

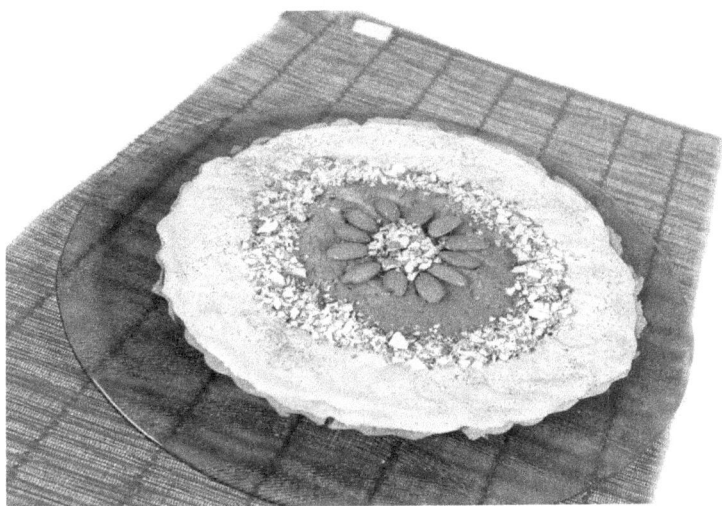

Raw Mango Pudding

2 Mangos
1 Cup of macadamia nuts soaked for 4 hours
1 Cup young coconut meat
1/8 Cup of lime juice
Shredded Coconut & Chopped macadamia nuts for the topping.

Use a vegetable peeler to peel mangos. Then cut the mango into pieces throwing away the pit. Drain the macadamia nuts and put all the ingredients in a blender and blend until smooth. Then add shredded coconut and chopped macadamia to taste.

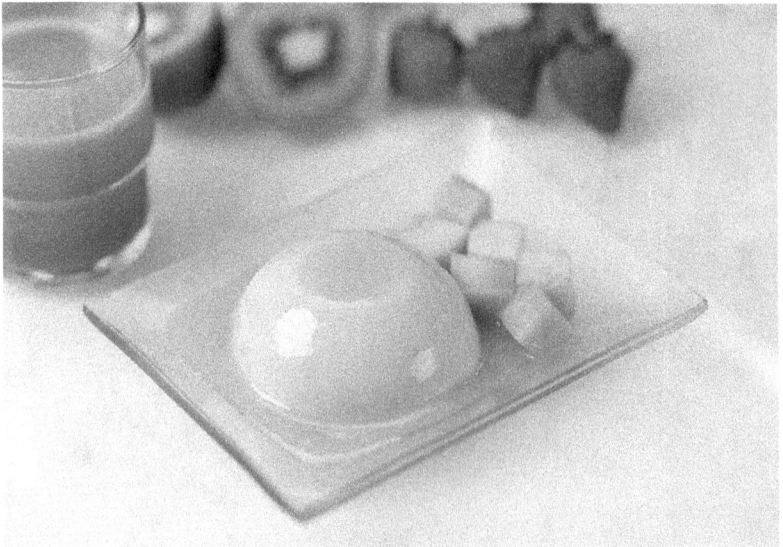

Raw Banana Coconut Cream Pie

For the Crust:

1 Cup Macadamia Nuts
½ Cup Shredded Dry Coconut
1 tsp Coconut Oil
2 Tablespoons of Raw Honey
Pinch of Salt

For the Filling:

2 Cups Young Coconut Meat About 2 young coconuts
½ Cup Raw Coconut Oil
3 Tablespoons of Raw Honey
2 Tablespoon Lime Juice
¼ teaspoon Salt
½ teaspoon Vanilla Extract
3 bananas (2 of them sliced)

Preparing The Crust
Blend first 5 ingredients in a food processor then add more honey if needed to make crust sticky. Line pie pan with saran wrap and press crust on top. Place in freezer while making the filling.

Preparing the Filling
Blend the rest of the ingredients, (**except bananas that are sliced**) in a vita mixer until smooth.

Make sure there is enough liquid to have the ingredients moving, you may need to add coconut water. Take crust out from freezer and place sliced bananas on top of crust. Pour filling on top of bananas. Place in freezer for 3-4 hours to set. Top with shredded coconut! Yum!

Raw "Chocolate Chip" Cookies

1 cup raw walnuts
1 Cup Pecans
1 Cup Macadamia Nuts
15 dates
1 Teaspoon of cinnamon
$\frac{1}{2}$ tsp salt
2 Tablespoon raw coconut oil
4 tablespoons cacao nibs

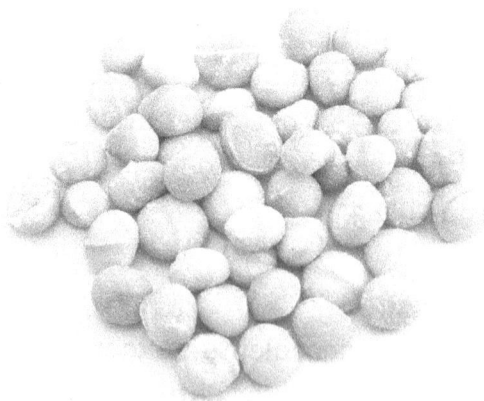

Place dates in food processor and mix until smooth. Add nuts, cinnamon, salt and coconut oil and mix it all up, again until smooth. Once smooth, add cacao nibs and blend just until nibs are well distributed. After ingredients are mixed, remove from food processor and use a spoon to make flat cookie shapes. Refrigerate before eating.

Raw Pecan Pie

For the crust:

1 Cup Macadamia Nuts
½ Cup Shredded Dry Coconut
1 tsp Coconut Oil
2 Tablespoons of Raw Honey
Pinch of Salt

For the filling:

3 cups pecans processed in a food processor until smooth
30 pitted dates
2 Cups shredded, dried coconut
1/2 teaspoon salt
1 teaspoon cinnamon
1/2 cup pecans, chopped

Preparing the Crust

Blend first 5 ingredients in a food
processor then add more honey if
needed to make crust sticky. Line pie
pan with saran wrap and press crust
on top. Place in freezer while making
the filling.

For the Filling:

In food processor, process dates until smooth (or as
close to smooth as you can get). Add the smooth pecans,
coconut, salt, and cinnamon. Process until everything is
well mixed. Remove from food processor and then place
ingredients in the prepared crust. Top with the extra
chopped pecans and then refrigerate for 1-2 hours.

Raw Chocolate Cream Pie

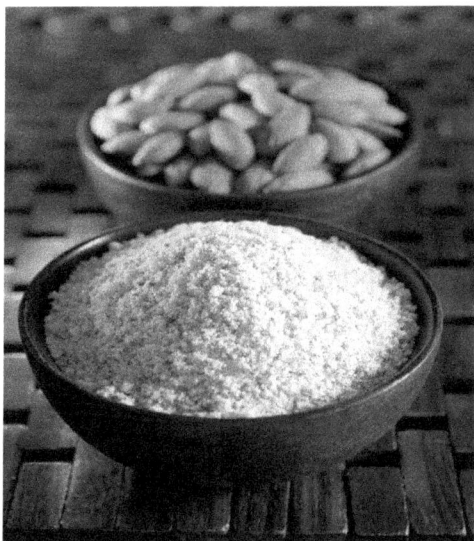

Crust
1/2 Cup Almonds
1/2 Cup Pecans
1/2 Cup of Brazil Nuts
 8 Pitted Dates
1/4 Cup Agave Syrup
1/4 Cup Cacao Powder
Pinch Sea Salt

Put nuts into food processor and process until ground.
Place the rest of the ingredients in processor with nuts
and process until combined. Spread onto a pie pan using
your hands.

Cream Filling
Meat of 2 Young Thai Coconuts
2 Avocado
6 Pitted Dates
1/2 Cup Cacao Powder
2 Tablespoons of Maple syrup

Place all ingredients in food processor and process until well combined. If filling is not sweet or chocolaty enough for you add a more syrup or more cacao powder respectively. Spread into inside of pie crust. Top with some sliced strawberries or raspberries for added flavor. Chill in refrigerator for 1-2 hours and serve.

Raw Apple Pie

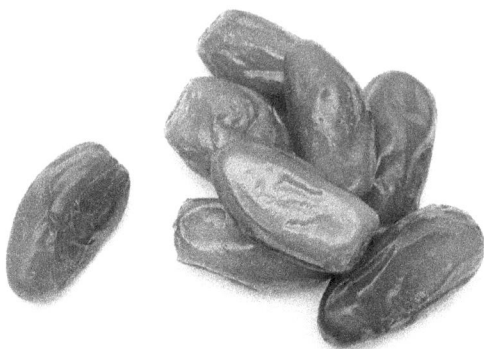

Crust:

1 ½ Cups of raw almonds soaked for 4-6 hours
1/8 Cup of Olive Oil
1 Tablespoon of coconut oil
Pinch of salt

Filling:

4-5 Red apples cored
5 Pitted dates
1 teaspoon of coconut oil
2 Tablespoons of maple syrup
1 teaspoon of cinnamon
Pinch of salt

Blend the almonds in a food processor and then add the rest of the crust ingredients. Put the crust into a glass pie pan. Next take the filling ingredients and blend

together and pour into the crust pan. Chill in the
refrigerator for 1-2 hours.

Raw Cheesecake

The Crust
2 Cups Raw macadamia nuts
8 Pitted dates
$\frac{1}{4}$ cup dried coconut

Filling:

3 Cups cashews soaked for at least 3 hours
$\frac{3}{4}$ Cup lemon juice
$\frac{3}{4}$ cups maple syrup
$\frac{3}{4}$ Cup coconut oil
Meat from one raw young coconut
$\frac{1}{2}$ cup cocoa nibs

Make the crust by processing the ingredients in a food
processor. Press the ingredients into a spring form pan.
Next blend the cashews, lemon, maple syrup, coconut oil,
young coconut meat, vanilla, and sea salt. Blend until
smooth. Pour the mixture onto the crust and top with
cocoa nibs and then freeze until firm.

Raw Banana & Chocolate Ice Cream

4 bananas sliced and then frozen
$\frac{1}{4}$ c raw cacao or cocoa powder
2 T raw honey
1 teaspoon vanilla
1 pinch of salt
$\frac{1}{4}$ cup cocoa nibs

Remove bananas from freezer and place them in a food processor; add cacao, honey, salt and vanilla and mix until thick and creamy. Add cocoa nibs and blend quickly, just until they are mixed through, but not ground too small. Pour mixture into a loaf pan and cover with saran wrap. Place in freezer. When serving, remove from freezer 5 minutes before. Scoop and serve, just as you would regular ice cream.

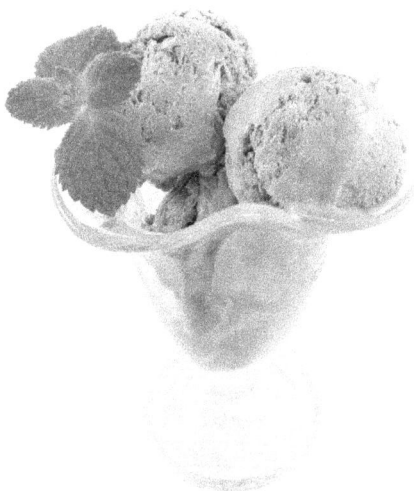

Rawberry Ice Cream

1 Frozen banana
1 Cup fresh strawberries
¼ Cup raw honey
The meat from one raw coconut
2 Cups raw cashews
Pinch of salt

Blend all ingredients in a food processor until smooth and then place in a container and freeze.

Raw Rice Pudding

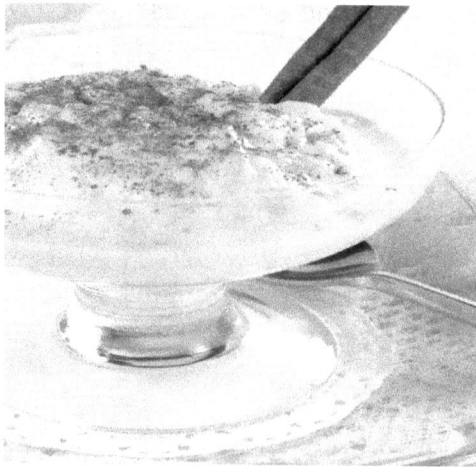

1 ½ Cup of brown rice soaked for 3 days
4 Young coconuts
2 teaspoons of cinnamon
1 teaspoon of nutmeg

1 teaspoon of vanilla
2 Tablespoons of maple syrup

In a vita mixer blend the coconut meat and only 2 cups of the coconut water, cinnamon, vanilla, and maple syrup. Blend until smooth. In a large bowl mix in the rice and the blended ingredients and let set in the refrigerator for 1 hour.

Chocolate Macadamia Pudding

2 Cups Raw macadamia nuts
2 Cups pitted dates
$\frac{1}{2}$ cup cocoa powder
1 Cup of coconut water

Blend all ingredients together until smooth and serve.

Raw Oatmeal Cookies

2 Cups Oats Soaked overnight
1/2 Cup of Almond milk
10 pitted dates
1 Cup of raw almonds
$\frac{1}{2}$ Cup Raisons
$\frac{1}{2}$ Cup Maple Syrup

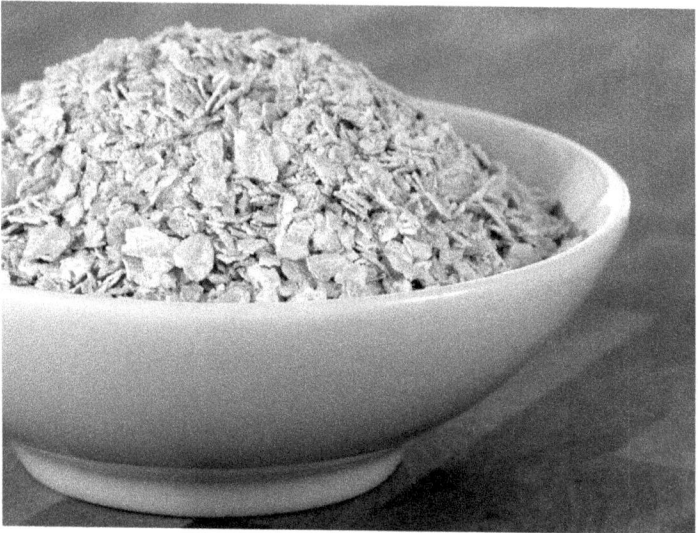

Mix all ingredients in a food processor (except the raisons) and blend. Next add the raisons. Now take small amounts of the dough and flatten on a dehydrator sheets so they resemble cookies and dehydrate for 12 hours at 110 degrees. Yum!

I hope you enjoy my raw dessert recipes!

You should check out some of my recipes at www.recipes4rawfood.com and www.rawfoodfortoday.com

I also wanted to include some very useful information on the benefits of nuts. Almost all of the desserts have nuts in them and I think that it would be good for you to know some of the benefits of the nuts for you and your family.

Benefits of Eating Raw Nuts

Nuts are an amazing food. Nuts are very beneficial for your health and they taste great too! Nuts are high in calories but they are still very beneficial to your body because they are loaded with mono saturated fats, which help to lower heart disease.   Many nuts are rich in omega 3 fatty acids. Omega 3 essential fatty acids are good for your heart and for your arteries. Omega 3 essential fatty acids are helpful for making your heart rhymes more stable so you can try to avoid a heart attack. Nuts also have L-arginine which is helpful to your heart and arteries because it makes your arteries more flexible and leads to less blood clots. Nuts also have been known to have plant sterols in them which help to lower cholesterol.

It is best to eat nuts raw, soaked, or sprouted because they are considered to be live foods. Live foods are foods that have not been heated at high temperatures or cooked. Heating nuts to above 118 degrees starts to destroy beneficial enzymes. When these enzymes are destroyed the nuts are unable to sprout so they would be considered not live.

Some of the best raw nuts are walnuts, cashews, brazil, macadamia, almonds, pecans, and filberts. They also make great milks when processed correctly. Almonds are one of my favorite nuts they are high in protein, vitamin E, magnesium, zinc, potassium, and iron. Almonds also have the highest amount of calcium of any other nut so they make a great substitute for dairy products for raw foodist and vegans. Almonds also have some of the highest fiber content of any other nut. Cashews are another good nut but should be refrigerated once the package is opened because the spoil easily. Cashews are high in copper and magnesium. Cashews also have one of the lowest fat content of any other nut. Macadamia nuts are also one of my favorites. Macadamia nuts are a high energy food and contain no cholesterol. The natural oils in macadamias contain 78% monounsaturated fats, the highest of any oil including olive oil. Macadamias contain tocopherols and tocotrienols, which are derivatives of Vitamin E, phytosterols such as sitosterol and also selenium. One of the best nuts for your health are walnuts. Walnuts are one of the best sources of omega 3 essential fatty acids and they have more antioxidants than most other nuts. Brazil nuts are extremely nutrient rich and high in antioxidants like selenium which helps to neutralize free radicals. Filberts are also very beneficial. If you add filberts to your salads or smoothies then they help you to absorb the fat soluble vitamins A, D, E, and K. Filberts are also great for anti aging properties such as Alzheimer's, stroke, arthritis, wrinkles, and heart disease.

Almost all nuts have photo nutrients which are biologically active components that protect our bodies systems. Many nuts act as antioxidants, which scavenge the free radicals that oxidize blood fats. Photo nutrients operate as part of complex systems that are only partly understood.

Nuts are an amazing food! They are so good for you and they taste great and can be used in so many raw and vegan recipes but just be careful to not over eat them because they are high in calories.

About the author

B.S. Science in Physical Anthropology minor in business, and Culinary Arts Degree. Advocate for organic, vegetarian, vegan, raw food diets, writing, yoga, swimming, biking, and running 5 K's!

I have been a vegetarian/vegan/raw foodist for over 20 years. I have also worked in real estate for over ten years and have several websites to help people who are interested in raw food www.Recipes4RawFood.com and www.RawFoodForToday.com.

I have also started the Raw Foods Association with my husband so that others can become members of a larger healthy group. For more information on how to become a member the website is www.RawFoodsAssociation.com!

For more information on how to order books, original articles, become a member of the Raw Foods Association, and updates on future projects go to www.rawfoodfortoday.com or www.recipes4rawfood.com.

Recipes 4 Raw Food
1314 E Las Olas Blvd
Fort Lauderdale, FL 33301

Recipes4rawfood@yahoo.com

www.ingramcontent.com/pod-product-compliance
Lightning Source LLC
Chambersburg PA
CBHW060703280326
41933CB00012B/2277